FATTY LIVER DIET COOKBOOK 2024:

Delicious and Nutritious Recipes to Revitalise, Detoxify and Aid Weight Loss

BY

LEE LAWRENCE

TABLE OF CONTENTS

INTRODUCTION

In the midst of our bustling modern lives, we often overlook one of the most vital organs in our body: the liver. Quietly toiling away, this unsung hero plays a crucial role in our overall health and well-being. Yet, due to the rapid pace of our lifestyles and the prevalence of processed foods, our livers can sometimes become burdened, leading to a condition known as fatty liver disease.

Fatty liver disease is a silent epidemic affecting millions worldwide, often without clear symptoms until it progresses to a more severe stage. It's a condition that demands attention and care, requiring us to rethink our dietary choices and lifestyle habits. But fear not, for within the pages of this book lies a transformative journey towards reclaiming control over your liver health and revitalizing your overall wellness.

Welcome to a culinary adventure like no other, where the power of wholesome ingredients and delicious flavors converge to create a symphony of nourishment and healing. Within these recipes, meticulously crafted and thoughtfully curated, lies the key to unlocking the potential of your liver to thrive once more.

In this cookbook, you'll embark on a journey through a treasure trove of quick and delectable recipes, each meticulously designed to not only tantalize your taste buds but also to nourish your body from within. From vibrant salads bursting with nutrients to hearty mains that will leave you feeling satisfied and energized, every dish is a testament to the idea that eating well is not just about sustenance—it's a celebration of life itself.

But this book is more than just a collection of recipes; it's a roadmap to a healthier, happier you. Within these pages, you'll find expert insights into the science behind liver health, empowering you with the knowledge to make informed choices about what you put on your plate. You'll discover the transformative power of ingredients carefully selected to support liver function and aid in detoxification, all without sacrificing flavor or enjoyment.

Whether you're embarking on a journey to reverse the effects of fatty liver disease, seeking to support your liver health preventatively, or simply looking to embrace a lifestyle of vitality and wellness, this book is your indispensable companion. It's a testament to the idea that nourishing your body can be both a pleasure and a privilege—a journey worth savoring with every bite.

So, as you turn the pages and embark on this culinary odyssey, remember that you hold in your hands not just a cookbook, but a roadmap to a healthier, happier you. Let the flavors guide you, the ingredients inspire you, and the joy of nourishment propel you forward on your journey towards optimal liver health and well-being. Welcome to a world where every meal is a step towards vitality, where food is not just sustenance, but a celebration of life itself.

CHAPTER 1: UNDERSTANDING FATTY LIVER DISEASE

What is Fatty Liver?

In recent years, fatty liver disease has become increasingly prevalent, emerging as a significant health concern worldwide. Understanding this condition is crucial for individuals to recognize its symptoms, manage its effects, and mitigate its progression. In this comprehensive guide, we delve into the intricacies of fatty liver disease, exploring its causes, symptoms, diagnosis, treatment options, and prevention strategies.

What is Fatty Liver?

Fatty liver disease, also known as hepatic steatosis, refers to the accumulation of excess fat in the liver. Normally, a small amount of fat is present in the liver. However, when fat accounts for more than 5-10% of the liver's weight, it is considered fatty liver disease. This condition can manifest in two main forms:

Non-alcoholic Fatty Liver Disease (NAFLD): This type of fatty liver disease occurs in individuals who consume little to no alcohol. It is often associated with obesity, insulin resistance, metabolic syndrome, and high levels of fats in the blood.

Alcoholic Fatty Liver Disease (AFLD): AFLD develops due to excessive alcohol consumption. It is the earliest stage of alcohol-related liver disease and can progress to more severe conditions such as alcoholic hepatitis and cirrhosis if alcohol consumption continues unabated.

Causes of Fatty Liver:

Several factors contribute to the development of fatty liver disease, including:

Obesity: Excess body weight, particularly visceral fat around the abdomen, increases the risk of fatty liver disease.

Insulin Resistance: Insulin resistance, a condition in which cells fail to respond adequately to insulin, is closely linked to the development of NAFLD.

Type 2 Diabetes: Individuals with diabetes are at an increased risk of developing NAFLD due to insulin resistance and metabolic abnormalities.

High Blood Lipids: Elevated levels of triglycerides and other fats in the blood can contribute to the accumulation of fat in the liver.

Excessive Alcohol Consumption: Chronic alcohol abuse is a leading cause of alcoholic fatty liver disease.

Symptoms of Fatty Liver:

Fatty liver disease is often asymptomatic in its early stages. However, as the condition progresses, individuals may experience symptoms such as:

- Fatigue
- Weakness
- Abdominal discomfort or pain in the upper right portion of the abdomen
- Enlarged liver
- Jaundice (yellowing of the skin and eyes) in severe cases

It's important to note that many of these symptoms are nonspecific and can be attributed to various other health conditions. Therefore, proper diagnosis by a healthcare professional is essential.

Diagnosis:

Diagnosing fatty liver disease typically involves a combination of medical history assessment, physical examination, and diagnostic tests, including:

Blood tests to assess liver function and levels of liver enzymes

Imaging studies such as ultrasound, CT scan, or MRI to visualize the liver and detect fat accumulation

Liver biopsy, in which a small sample of liver tissue is removed and examined under a microscope to confirm the diagnosis and assess the degree of liver damage

Treatment Options:

The treatment approach for fatty liver disease focuses on addressing underlying risk factors and preventing further liver damage. Treatment strategies may include:

Lifestyle Modifications: Adopting a healthy lifestyle is crucial for managing fatty liver disease. This includes maintaining a balanced diet, achieving and maintaining a healthy weight, engaging in regular physical activity, and avoiding excessive alcohol consumption. Medications: In some cases, medications may be prescribed to help control underlying conditions such as diabetes, high cholesterol, or metabolic syndrome.

Follow-up Care: Regular monitoring and follow-up with healthcare providers are essential

to assess liver function, monitor disease progression, and adjust treatment as needed.
Prevention Strategies:

Preventing fatty liver disease involves adopting healthy lifestyle habits and minimizing risk factors. Key preventive measures include:

Maintaining a healthy weight through a balanced diet and regular exercise
Limiting alcohol consumption to moderate levels or abstaining from alcohol altogether
Managing underlying conditions such as diabetes, high cholesterol, and hypertension
Avoiding crash diets or rapid weight loss regimens that can exacerbate liver damage

Fatty liver disease is a common yet potentially serious condition that requires attention and proactive management. By understanding its causes, symptoms, diagnosis, and treatment options, individuals can take proactive steps to protect their liver health and reduce the risk of complications. Consulting with healthcare professionals and adopting a healthy lifestyle are essential components of managing fatty liver disease and promoting overall well-being.

Causes and Risk Factors

Fatty liver disease, also known as hepatic steatosis, is a condition characterized by the accumulation of fat in the liver cells. It is a growing health concern globally, with its prevalence increasing due to rising rates of obesity, sedentary lifestyles, and poor dietary habits. Understanding the causes and risk factors associated with fatty liver disease is crucial for prevention, early detection, and effective management of this condition.

Causes of Fatty Liver Disease:

Obesity: Excess body weight, especially abdominal obesity, is strongly linked to the development of fatty liver disease. The accumulation of visceral fat can lead to insulin resistance and increased fat deposition in the liver.

Insulin Resistance: Insulin is a hormone that regulates blood sugar levels. Insulin resistance occurs when cells in the body become resistant to the effects of insulin, leading to higher blood sugar levels. This can trigger the liver to store more fat, contributing to fatty liver disease.

Type 2 Diabetes: People with type 2 diabetes are at an increased risk of developing fatty liver disease due to insulin resistance and elevated levels of circulating fats in the blood.

High Blood Sugar Levels: Chronic high blood sugar levels, as seen in diabetes or prediabetes, can promote fat accumulation in the liver.

Unhealthy Diet: Consuming a diet high in calories, particularly from sugars and unhealthy fats, can contribute to the development of fatty liver disease. Excessive intake of processed foods, sugary beverages, and trans fats can overload the liver's ability to metabolize fats efficiently.

High Levels of Triglycerides: Elevated levels of triglycerides, a type of fat found in the blood, can increase the risk of fatty liver disease. This often occurs in individuals with obesity, insulin resistance, or metabolic syndrome.

Alcohol Consumption: Excessive alcohol consumption is a common cause of fatty liver disease. Alcohol is metabolized by the liver, and chronic alcohol abuse can lead to inflammation and fatty deposits in the liver cells.

Risk Factors for Fatty Liver Disease:

Obesity: Being overweight or obese significantly increases the risk of fatty liver disease. Excess adipose tissue, especially around the abdomen, is closely associated with insulin resistance and fatty liver development.

Type 2 Diabetes: Individuals with type 2 diabetes are at a higher risk of developing fatty liver disease due to insulin resistance and dysregulated lipid metabolism.

Metabolic Syndrome: Metabolic syndrome is a cluster of conditions including obesity, high blood pressure, high blood sugar, and abnormal lipid levels. It greatly increases the risk of fatty liver disease.

Insulin Resistance: Insulin resistance, commonly associated with obesity and type 2 diabetes, is a key risk factor for fatty liver disease.

High Cholesterol and Triglycerides: Elevated levels of cholesterol and triglycerides in the blood are associated with an increased risk of fatty liver disease.

Poor Dietary Habits: A diet high in refined carbohydrates, sugars, and unhealthy fats contributes to the development of fatty liver disease.

Sedentary Lifestyle: Lack of physical activity is linked to obesity, insulin resistance, and other risk factors for fatty liver disease.

Family History: A family history of fatty liver disease or related conditions such as type 2 diabetes and cardiovascular disease may increase an individual's susceptibility to the condition.

Fatty liver disease is a complex condition influenced by various genetic, lifestyle, and environmental factors. While it is often asymptomatic in the early stages, it can progress to more severe liver damage if left untreated. Prevention and management strategies focus on lifestyle modifications such as maintaining a healthy weight, following a balanced diet, engaging in regular physical activity, limiting alcohol consumption, and managing underlying health conditions like diabetes and high cholesterol. Understanding the causes and risk factors associated with fatty liver disease is essential for promoting liver health and reducing the burden of this increasingly prevalent condition.

Effects on Health

Fatty liver disease, also known as hepatic steatosis, is a prevalent yet often misunderstood condition affecting millions of people worldwide. Characterized by the accumulation of fat in liver cells, this disease can have significant implications for one's health and well-being. Understanding its causes, symptoms, and effects on health is crucial for effective management and prevention.

Causes of Fatty Liver Disease:

Non-Alcoholic Fatty Liver Disease (NAFLD): This is the most common form of fatty liver disease, often associated with obesity, insulin resistance, high cholesterol, and metabolic syndrome.

Alcoholic Fatty Liver Disease (AFLD): As the name suggests, this type is caused by excessive alcohol consumption, which leads to fat buildup in the liver.

Other Causes: Certain medications, rapid weight loss, viral hepatitis, and genetic factors can also contribute to fatty liver disease.

Symptoms of Fatty Liver Disease:

Fatty liver disease is often asymptomatic in its early stages. However, as the condition progresses, individuals may experience:

- Fatigue
- Abdominal discomfort or pain
- Jaundice (yellowing of the skin and eyes)
- Swelling in the abdomen or legs
- Loss of appetite

- Unintended weight loss

Effects on Health:

Liver Inflammation (Steatohepatitis): In some cases, fatty liver disease can progress to steatohepatitis, which involves liver inflammation. This can lead to liver cell damage and scarring (cirrhosis), impairing liver function over time.

Increased Risk of Liver Cancer: Individuals with fatty liver disease, especially those with advanced stages or cirrhosis, have a higher risk of developing liver cancer (hepatocellular carcinoma).

Cardiovascular Complications: Fatty liver disease is often associated with other metabolic conditions such as obesity, diabetes, and high cholesterol, increasing the risk of cardiovascular diseases such as heart attacks and strokes.

Insulin Resistance and Diabetes: NAFLD is closely linked to insulin resistance, a condition where the body's cells become resistant to the effects of insulin. This can lead to type 2 diabetes if left unmanaged.

Complications During Surgery: Fatty liver disease, particularly in its advanced stages, can pose challenges during surgical procedures due to impaired liver function and increased bleeding risk.

Diagnosis and Management:

Physical Examination: Your doctor may perform a physical exam and inquire about your medical history and lifestyle habits.

Blood Tests: Blood tests can assess liver function and check for elevated liver enzymes, indicating liver damage.

Imaging Studies: Ultrasound, CT scans, or MRI scans can visualize fat accumulation in the liver.

Liver Biopsy: In some cases, a liver biopsy may be necessary to confirm the diagnosis and assess the degree of liver damage.

Lifestyle Modifications: Management typically involves lifestyle changes such as weight loss, adopting a balanced diet, regular exercise, limiting alcohol consumption, and avoiding unnecessary medications.

Medications: In certain cases, medications may be prescribed to manage underlying conditions such as diabetes, high cholesterol, or to reduce liver inflammation.

Monitoring and Follow-Up: Regular monitoring and follow-up with healthcare providers are essential to track the progression of the disease and adjust treatment strategies accordingly.

Prevention:

Maintaining a healthy weight through diet and exercise.

Limiting alcohol consumption.

Avoiding rapid weight loss or crash diets.

Monitoring and managing underlying health conditions such as diabetes and high cholesterol.

Regularly screening for liver function and fatty liver disease risk factors.

:

Fatty liver disease is a common yet potentially serious condition that requires attention and proactive management. By understanding its causes, symptoms, and effects on health, individuals can take steps to prevent or mitigate its progression. Early diagnosis, lifestyle modifications, and appropriate medical care play pivotal roles in managing fatty liver disease and reducing its impact on overall health and well-being.

CHAPTER 2: BASICS OF FATTY LIVER DIET

Importance of Diet in Managing Fatty Liver

In the modern era of sedentary lifestyles and processed food abundance, fatty liver disease has become increasingly prevalent. Characterized by the accumulation of fat in liver cells, this condition can lead to inflammation, scarring, and ultimately, liver damage. However, there's a glimmer of hope amidst this health concern: diet. The significance of dietary choices in managing fatty liver cannot be overstated. By adopting a well-rounded, nourishing diet, individuals can alleviate symptoms, improve liver health, and foster overall well-being. Let's delve into the fundamental principles of a fatty liver diet and understand its pivotal role in combating this condition.

Understanding Fatty Liver Disease:

Before diving into dietary specifics, it's essential to grasp the basics of fatty liver disease. Typically, there are two primary types: alcoholic fatty liver disease (AFLD) and non-alcoholic fatty liver disease (NAFLD). AFLD stems from excessive alcohol consumption, while NAFLD is associated with factors such as obesity, insulin resistance, and metabolic syndrome. Regardless of the type, dietary interventions play a crucial role in managing both conditions.

The Importance of Diet:

The liver is a metabolic powerhouse responsible for numerous vital functions, including detoxification, nutrient processing, and bile production. When excess fat accumulates in liver cells, it compromises these functions, leading to inflammation and potential damage. A strategic dietary approach aims to reduce fat deposition, ease liver burden, and promote regeneration. Moreover, dietary modifications can address underlying factors like obesity and insulin resistance, which often accompany fatty liver disease.

Key Principles of a Fatty Liver Diet:

Limit Saturated Fats and Trans Fats: These unhealthy fats contribute to lipid accumulation in the liver. Opt for healthier fats like those found in nuts, seeds, avocados, and fatty fish such as salmon and mackerel.

Embrace Whole Foods: Base your diet on whole, unprocessed foods such as fruits, vegetables, whole grains, and lean proteins. These nutrient-dense choices provide essential vitamins, minerals, and antioxidants, supporting liver health and overall vitality.

Control Portion Sizes and Calories: Excess calorie intake, particularly from refined sugars and carbohydrates, can exacerbate fatty liver disease. Practice portion control and opt for low-glycemic index carbohydrates to stabilize blood sugar levels.

Prioritize Fiber: Dietary fiber aids digestion, promotes satiety, and helps regulate blood sugar and cholesterol levels. Incorporate plenty of fiber-rich foods like legumes, oats, vegetables, and fruits into your meals.

Moderate Alcohol Consumption: For individuals with AFLD or NAFLD, reducing or eliminating alcohol consumption is paramount. Alcohol not only contributes to liver inflammation but also exacerbates existing liver damage.

Stay Hydrated: Adequate hydration supports liver function and helps flush toxins from the body. Aim to drink plenty of water throughout the day, and limit sugary beverages and excessive caffeine intake.

Include Liver-Supportive Nutrients: Certain nutrients are particularly beneficial for liver health, including vitamin E, vitamin C, selenium, and antioxidants like glutathione. These can be obtained from a variety of foods, including nuts, seeds, leafy greens, citrus fruits, and lean meats.

Seek Professional Guidance: Every individual's nutritional needs are unique, and dietary recommendations should be tailored to specific health conditions and goals. Consulting with a registered dietitian or healthcare provider can provide personalized guidance and support.

In the journey to manage fatty liver disease, diet serves as a cornerstone of treatment and prevention. By adopting a balanced, nutrient-rich eating pattern and making mindful lifestyle choices, individuals can support liver health, reduce inflammation, and improve overall quality of life. Remember, small dietary changes can yield significant benefits over time, empowering individuals to take charge of their health and well-being.

Foods to Include and Avoid

Fatty liver disease is becoming increasingly prevalent, affecting millions of people worldwide. It's a condition where excess fat accumulates in the liver, leading to inflammation and potential damage if left unaddressed. While various factors contribute to fatty liver disease, including genetics and lifestyle choices, diet plays a crucial role in both prevention and management. Adopting a fatty liver diet can help reduce fat buildup, promote liver health, and prevent complications. Let's delve into the fundamentals of a fatty liver diet, including foods to include and avoid.

Foods to Include:

Fruits and Vegetables: Incorporate a variety of colorful fruits and vegetables into your diet. These are rich in antioxidants, vitamins, and minerals, which help reduce inflammation and protect liver cells from damage. Opt for options like berries, citrus fruits, leafy greens, broccoli, and bell peppers.

Whole Grains: Choose whole grains over refined grains to increase fiber intake and promote satiety. Whole grains like oats, quinoa, brown rice, and whole wheat bread provide essential nutrients and help regulate blood sugar levels, reducing the risk of insulin resistance associated with fatty liver disease.

Lean Protein Sources: Include lean sources of protein such as poultry, fish, tofu, legumes, and eggs in your diet. These provide amino acids necessary for liver repair and maintenance without adding excessive saturated fats.

Healthy Fats: Incorporate healthy fats like those found in avocados, nuts, seeds, and olive oil. These fats contain omega-3 fatty acids and monounsaturated fats, which have anti-inflammatory properties and support overall liver function.

Low-Fat Dairy: Opt for low-fat or skim dairy products to reduce saturated fat intake while still obtaining essential nutrients like calcium and vitamin D. Choose options like skim milk, yogurt, and cheese in moderation.

Herbs and Spices: Enhance the flavor of your meals with herbs and spices like turmeric, ginger, cinnamon, and garlic. These ingredients not only add zest to your dishes but also possess anti-inflammatory properties beneficial for liver health.

Foods to Avoid:

Sugary Foods and Beverages: Minimize consumption of sugary foods and beverages, including soda, candy, pastries, and processed snacks. Excess sugar consumption can contribute to insulin resistance and exacerbate fatty liver disease.

Highly Processed Foods: Steer clear of highly processed foods high in unhealthy fats, refined carbohydrates, and additives. These include fast food, fried foods, packaged snacks, and sugary cereals, which can contribute to liver inflammation and weight gain.

Alcohol: Limit or eliminate alcohol consumption as it can significantly worsen fatty liver disease. Alcohol is metabolized by the liver, leading to the accumulation of fat and inflammation. Even moderate alcohol consumption can be detrimental to liver health.

Saturated and Trans Fats: Reduce intake of saturated and trans fats found in red meat, fatty cuts of meat, butter, margarine, and processed foods. These fats can raise cholesterol levels and contribute to liver damage.

Excessive Salt: Limit sodium intake to prevent fluid retention and reduce the risk of complications such as ascites. Avoid high-sodium processed foods, canned soups, and salty snacks.

High Cholesterol Foods: Avoid foods high in cholesterol, such as organ meats, shellfish, and full-fat dairy products. High cholesterol levels can exacerbate fatty liver disease and increase the risk of cardiovascular complications.

A well-planned fatty liver diet plays a pivotal role in managing and preventing the progression of fatty liver disease. By focusing on nutrient-dense foods, limiting harmful dietary components, and maintaining a balanced lifestyle, individuals can support liver health and reduce the risk of complications. However, it's essential to consult with a healthcare professional or a registered dietitian before making significant dietary changes, especially if you have underlying health conditions or are taking medications. With dedication and commitment to a healthy lifestyle, individuals can take control of their liver health and improve overall well-being.

Lifestyle Changes for Liver Health

Maintaining a healthy liver is crucial for overall well-being. Fatty liver disease, characterized by the accumulation of fat in liver cells, is becoming increasingly common due to sedentary lifestyles and poor dietary habits. Fortunately, adopting a fatty liver diet and making lifestyle changes can help manage this condition effectively. In this guide, we'll explore the fundamentals of a fatty liver diet and lifestyle modifications to support liver health.

Understanding Fatty Liver Disease:

Before diving into dietary and lifestyle recommendations, it's essential to understand fatty liver disease. There are two primary types: alcoholic fatty liver disease (AFLD) and non-alcoholic fatty liver disease (NAFLD). AFLD occurs due to excessive alcohol consumption, while NAFLD is associated with factors like obesity, insulin resistance, and high cholesterol. Both can progress to more severe conditions like liver cirrhosis and liver failure if left untreated.

Basics of a Fatty Liver Diet:

Emphasize Whole Foods: Focus on incorporating whole, unprocessed foods into your diet. These include fruits, vegetables, lean proteins, whole grains, and healthy fats like those found in avocados, nuts, and olive oil. These foods provide essential nutrients and antioxidants that support liver function and reduce inflammation.

Limit Saturated Fats and Sugars: Reduce your intake of saturated fats found in red meat, fried foods, and full-fat dairy products. Additionally, cut back on added sugars and refined carbohydrates, as they can contribute to insulin resistance and liver fat accumulation.

Choose Healthy Proteins: Opt for lean protein sources such as poultry, fish, tofu, legumes, and low-fat dairy. These protein sources provide amino acids necessary for liver repair and regeneration without adding excess fat to the diet.

Monitor Portion Sizes: Be mindful of portion sizes to prevent overeating, which can lead to weight gain and exacerbate fatty liver disease. Focus on eating smaller, more frequent meals throughout the day to help stabilize blood sugar levels and prevent excessive fat accumulation in the liver.

Stay Hydrated: Drink plenty of water throughout the day to support liver function and facilitate the elimination of toxins from the body. Limit consumption of sugary beverages and alcohol, as they can contribute to liver damage and dehydration.

Lifestyle Changes for Liver Health:

Regular Exercise: Engage in regular physical activity to promote weight loss, improve insulin sensitivity, and reduce liver fat. Aim for at least 30 minutes of moderate-intensity exercise most days of the week, such as brisk walking, cycling, swimming, or strength training.

Manage Stress: Chronic stress can negatively impact liver health by triggering inflammation and promoting unhealthy coping mechanisms like overeating or excessive alcohol consumption. Practice stress-reducing techniques such as meditation, deep breathing exercises, yoga, or spending time in nature to promote relaxation and emotional well-being.

Get Adequate Sleep: Prioritize quality sleep, as inadequate sleep patterns have been linked to liver disease progression. Aim for 7-9 hours of uninterrupted sleep per night, and establish a consistent sleep schedule to support optimal liver function and overall health.

Avoid Harmful Substances: Minimize exposure to toxins and harmful substances that can strain the liver, such as cigarette smoke, environmental pollutants, and excessive alcohol consumption. Quit smoking if you smoke, and limit alcohol intake to moderate levels or abstain altogether if advised by a healthcare professional.

Regular Monitoring: Regularly monitor your liver health through routine medical check-ups and screenings. If diagnosed with fatty liver disease, work closely with your healthcare provider to develop a personalized treatment plan tailored to your specific needs and goals.

Adopting a fatty liver diet and making lifestyle changes are essential steps in managing fatty liver disease and promoting overall liver health. By prioritizing nutrient-dense foods, regular exercise, stress management, adequate sleep, and avoiding harmful substances, you can support your liver's natural detoxification processes and reduce the risk of disease progression. Remember to consult with a healthcare professional before making significant dietary or lifestyle changes, especially if you have existing health conditions or are taking medications. With dedication and commitment, you can nourish your liver and enjoy improved health and vitality.

CHAPTER 3: BREAKFAST DELIGHTS

Avocado and Spinach Omelette

Cooking Time: 10 minutes

Serving Time: Immediate

Total Time: 10 minutes

Ingredients:

- 2 eggs
- 1/4 cup chopped spinach
- 1/4 avocado, sliced
- Salt and pepper to taste
- 1 tablespoon olive oil

Directions:

- Heat olive oil in a non-stick skillet over medium heat.

- In a bowl, beat eggs and season with salt and pepper.

- Pour eggs into the skillet and let them cook for 1-2 minutes until the edges start to set.

- Sprinkle chopped spinach over half of the omelette.

- When the omelette is mostly set, fold it in half with a spatula.

- Cook for another 2-3 minutes until fully cooked.

- Slide onto a plate and top with sliced avocado.

- Serve immediately.

Tips:

- Be gentle when folding the omelette to prevent it from breaking.
- You can add cheese or other vegetables for extra flavor.

Quinoa Breakfast Bowl

Cooking Time: 15 minutes

Serving Time: Immediate

Total Time: 15 minutes

Ingredients:

- 1/2 cup cooked quinoa
- 1/4 cup almond milk
- 1 tablespoon honey
- 1/2 banana, sliced
- 1/4 cup mixed berries
- 1 tablespoon chopped nuts (e.g., almonds, walnuts)

Directions:

- In a small saucepan, warm cooked quinoa with almond milk over medium heat.
- Stir in honey until well combined.

- Transfer the quinoa mixture to a bowl.

- Top with sliced banana, mixed berries, and chopped nuts.

- Serve immediately.

Tips:

- You can customize the toppings with your favorite fruits and nuts.

- Adjust sweetness by adding more or less honey according to your taste.

Chia Seed Pudding with Berries

Preparation Time: 5 minutes

Chilling Time: 2 hours

Serving Time: Immediate

Total Time: 2 hours 5 minutes

Ingredients:

- 2 tablespoons chia seeds
- 1/2 cup almond milk
- 1 tablespoon honey
- 1/4 cup mixed berries

Directions:

- In a bowl, mix chia seeds, almond milk, and honey.
- Stir well and let it sit for 5 minutes.
- Stir again to break up any clumps of chia seeds.

- Cover the bowl and refrigerate for at least 2 hours or overnight.
- Once chilled, stir the pudding and transfer it to serving bowls.
- Top with mixed berries before serving.

Tips:

- You can prepare the pudding the night before for a quick breakfast.
- Experiment with different toppings like sliced bananas or shredded coconut.

Greek Yogurt Parfait

Assembly Time: 5 minutes

Serving Time: Immediate

Total Time: 5 minutes

Ingredients:

- 1/2 cup Greek yogurt
- 1/4 cup granola
- 1/4 cup mixed berries
- Honey for drizzling

Directions:

- In a glass or bowl, layer Greek yogurt, granola, and mixed berries.
- Repeat layers until the glass is filled.
- Drizzle honey on top.
- Serve immediately.

Tips:

- Use plain Greek yogurt for a healthier option.
- Make it ahead of time and keep it refrigerated until ready to serve.

Smoked Salmon and Avocado Toast

Preparation Time: 5 minutes

Cooking Time: 5 minutes

Serving Time: Immediate

Total Time: 10 minutes

Ingredients:

- 2 slices whole grain bread
- 1/2 avocado, mashed
- 2 ounces smoked salmon
- Lemon juice (optional)
- Salt and pepper to taste
- Fresh dill or chives for garnish (optional)

Directions:

- Toast the bread slices until golden brown.
- Spread mashed avocado evenly on each slice.

- Arrange smoked salmon on top of the avocado.
- Squeeze lemon juice over the salmon if desired.
- Season with salt and pepper.
- Garnish with fresh dill or chives if using.
- Serve immediately.

Tips:

- Add a poached or fried egg on top for extra protein.
- Use a squeeze bottle for easy and precise lemon juice application.

Berry Blast Smoothie

Preparation Time: 5 minutes

Blending Time: 2 minutes

Serving Time: Immediate

Total Time: 7 minutes

Ingredients:

- 1 cup mixed berries (strawberries, blueberries, raspberries)
- 1/2 banana
- 1/2 cup Greek yogurt
- 1/2 cup almond milk
- 1 tablespoon honey or maple syrup (optional)
- Ice cubes (optional)

Directions:

- Place mixed berries, banana, Greek yogurt, almond milk, and honey or maple syrup (if using) in a blender.
- Blend until smooth.
- Add ice cubes if desired and blend again until well combined.
- Pour into glasses and serve immediately.

Tips:

- Adjust the sweetness by adding more or less honey according to your taste.
- Freeze the berries beforehand for a thicker consistency.

Veggie and Egg Muffin Cups

Preparation Time: 10 minutes

Baking Time: 20 minutes

Serving Time: Immediate

Total Time: 30 minutes

Ingredients:

- 6 eggs
- 1/4 cup chopped bell peppers
- 1/4 cup chopped spinach
- 1/4 cup shredded cheese
- Salt and pepper to taste

Directions:

- Preheat the oven to 350°F (175°C) and grease a muffin tin.
- In a bowl, whisk eggs and season with salt and pepper.

- Stir in chopped bell peppers, chopped spinach, and shredded cheese.
- Pour the egg mixture evenly into the muffin cups, filling each about 3/4 full.
- Bake for 20 minutes or until the eggs are set.
- Allow the muffins to cool for a few minutes before removing them from the tin.
- Serve warm.

Tips:

- You can customize the veggies and add cooked bacon or sausage for extra flavor.
- Store leftovers in an airtight container in the refrigerator for quick breakfasts during the week.

Banana Walnut Pancakes

Preparation Time: 10 minutes

Cooking Time: 10 minutes

Serving Time: Immediate

Total Time: 20 minutes

Ingredients:

- 1 cup all-purpose flour
- 1 tablespoon sugar
- 1 teaspoon baking powder
- 1/4 teaspoon salt
- 1 ripe banana, mashed
- 1 egg
- 3/4 cup milk
- 1/4 cup chopped walnuts
- Butter or oil for cooking

Directions:

- In a large bowl, whisk together flour, sugar, baking powder, and salt.
- In another bowl, mix mashed banana, egg, and milk until well combined.
- Pour the wet ingredients into the dry ingredients and stir until just combined.
- Fold in chopped walnuts.
- Heat a non-stick skillet or griddle over medium heat and lightly grease with butter or oil.
- Pour about 1/4 cup of batter onto the skillet for each pancake.
- Cook until bubbles form on the surface, then flip and cook until golden brown on the other side.
- Repeat with the remaining batter.

- Serve warm with maple syrup or your favorite toppings.

Tips:

- For extra flavor, add a dash of cinnamon or vanilla extract to the batter.
- Make a large batch and freeze the pancakes for future breakfasts. Simply reheat in the toaster or microwave.

CHAPTER 4: ENERGIZING LUNCHES

Grilled Chicken Salad with Lemon Dressing

Preparation Time: 10 minutes

Cooking Time: 10 minutes

Serving Time: Immediate

Total Time: 20 minutes

Ingredients:

- 2 boneless, skinless chicken breasts
- Salt and pepper to taste
- 4 cups mixed salad greens
- 1 cup cherry tomatoes, halved
- 1/2 cucumber, sliced
- 1/4 red onion, thinly sliced

- 1/4 cup feta cheese, crumbled (optional)

For Lemon Dressing:

- 1/4 cup olive oil
- 2 tablespoons lemon juice
- 1 teaspoon Dijon mustard
- 1 clove garlic, minced
- Salt and pepper to taste

Directions:

- Season chicken breasts with salt and pepper.
- Heat a grill pan or outdoor grill over medium-high heat.
- Grill chicken for 5-6 minutes on each side or until cooked through.
- Let the chicken rest for a few minutes before slicing.

- In a small bowl, whisk together olive oil, lemon juice, Dijon mustard, minced garlic, salt, and pepper to make the dressing.
- In a large bowl, toss mixed salad greens, cherry tomatoes, cucumber, and red onion with the lemon dressing.
- Divide the salad among plates and top with sliced grilled chicken.
- Optional: Sprinkle crumbled feta cheese over the salad.
- Serve immediately.

Tips:

- Marinate the chicken in the dressing for extra flavor before grilling.
- You can use leftover grilled chicken for this recipe to save time.

Lentil Soup with Turmeric

Preparation Time: 10 minutes

Cooking Time: 30 minutes

Serving Time: Immediate

Total Time: 40 minutes

Ingredients:

- 1 tablespoon olive oil
- 1 onion, diced
- 2 carrots, diced
- 2 celery stalks, diced
- 2 cloves garlic, minced
- 1 teaspoon ground turmeric
- 1 cup dried lentils, rinsed
- 4 cups vegetable broth
- Salt and pepper to taste
- Fresh parsley for garnish (optional)

Directions:

- Heat olive oil in a large pot over medium heat.
- Add diced onion, carrots, and celery. Cook until vegetables are softened, about 5 minutes.
- Stir in minced garlic and ground turmeric, and cook for another minute.
- Add dried lentils and vegetable broth to the pot.
- Bring the soup to a boil, then reduce heat to low and simmer for 20-25 minutes, or until lentils are tender.
- Season with salt and pepper to taste.
- Ladle the soup into bowls and garnish with fresh parsley if desired.
- Serve hot.

Tips:

- You can blend a portion of the soup for a creamier texture if desired.
- Add a squeeze of lemon juice before serving for extra freshness.

Zucchini Noodles with Pesto

Preparation Time: 10 minutes

Cooking Time: 5 minutes

Serving Time: Immediate

Total Time: 15 minutes

Ingredients:

- 2 medium zucchinis
- 1/4 cup basil pesto (store-bought or homemade)
- Cherry tomatoes, halved (optional)
- Grated Parmesan cheese for garnish (optional)

Directions:

- Use a spiralizer to create zucchini noodles.
- Heat a large skillet over medium heat.

- Add zucchini noodles to the skillet and cook for 2-3 minutes, tossing occasionally, until just tender.
- Transfer the cooked zucchini noodles to a serving dish.
- Toss the zucchini noodles with basil pesto until well coated.
- Optional: Add cherry tomatoes halves for extra flavor and color.
- Garnish with grated Parmesan cheese if desired.
- Serve immediately.

Tips:

- Be careful not to overcook the zucchini noodles to prevent them from becoming mushy.

- You can add grilled chicken or shrimp for additional protein.

Black Bean and Corn Quesadillas

Preparation Time: 10 minutes

Cooking Time: 10 minutes

Serving Time: Immediate

Total Time: 20 minutes

Ingredients:

- 4 medium flour tortillas
- 1 cup canned black beans, drained and rinsed
- 1 cup frozen corn, thawed
- 1 cup shredded cheese (cheddar, Monterey Jack, or Mexican blend)
- 1/2 teaspoon ground cumin
- 1/2 teaspoon chili powder
- Salt and pepper to taste
- Olive oil for cooking

Directions:

- In a bowl, mix black beans, corn, shredded cheese, ground cumin, chili powder, salt, and pepper.
- Heat a skillet over medium heat.
- Place a tortilla in the skillet and spoon a quarter of the bean and corn mixture onto one half of the tortilla.
- Fold the other half of the tortilla over the filling to create a half-moon shape.
- Cook for 2-3 minutes on each side until golden brown and crispy.
- Repeat with the remaining tortillas and filling.
- Cut each quesadilla into wedges and serve hot.

Tips:

- Customize with your favorite fillings like diced bell peppers, onions, or jalapeños.
- Serve with salsa, guacamole, or sour cream on the side.

Quinoa Stuffed Bell Peppers

Preparation Time: 15 minutes

Cooking Time: 30 minutes

Serving Time: Immediate

Total Time: 45 minutes

Ingredients:

- 4 large bell peppers, halved and seeds removed
- 1 cup cooked quinoa
- 1 cup black beans, drained and rinsed
- 1 cup diced tomatoes
- 1/2 cup corn kernels
- 1/2 cup shredded cheese (cheddar, mozzarella, or pepper jack)
- 1 teaspoon chili powder
- 1/2 teaspoon ground cumin
- Salt and pepper to taste

- Fresh cilantro for garnish (optional)

Directions:

- Preheat the oven to 375°F (190°C).
- In a large bowl, mix cooked quinoa, black beans, diced tomatoes, corn kernels, shredded cheese, chili powder, ground cumin, salt, and pepper.
- Stuff each bell pepper half with the quinoa mixture.
- Place stuffed bell peppers in a baking dish.
- Cover the dish with aluminum foil and bake for 25-30 minutes, or until the peppers are tender.
- Remove the foil and bake for an additional 5 minutes to melt the cheese.
- Garnish with fresh cilantro if desired.

- Serve hot.

Tips:

- Add cooked ground turkey or chicken to the quinoa mixture for extra protein.
- Make it vegan by omitting the cheese or using a vegan cheese alternative.

Tuna Salad Lettuce Wraps

Preparation Time: 10 minutes

Serving Time: Immediate

Total Time: 10 minutes

Ingredients:

- 2 cans (5 ounces each) tuna, drained
- 1/4 cup mayonnaise
- 2 tablespoons diced red onion
- 2 tablespoons diced celery
- 1 tablespoon lemon juice
- Salt and pepper to taste
- Lettuce leaves for wrapping
- Sliced avocado for topping (optional)
- Sliced cherry tomatoes for topping (optional)

Directions:

- In a bowl, combine drained tuna, mayonnaise, diced red onion, diced celery, lemon juice, salt, and pepper.
- Mix until well combined.
- Spoon tuna salad onto lettuce leaves.
- Top with sliced avocado and cherry tomatoes if desired.
- Wrap the lettuce around the filling.
- Serve immediately.

Tips:

- Use Greek yogurt instead of mayonnaise for a healthier alternative.
- Add diced pickles or relish for extra flavor and crunch.

Cauliflower Fried Rice

Preparation Time: 10 minutes

Cooking Time: 10 minutes

Serving Time: Immediate

Total Time: 20 minutes

Ingredients:

- 1 medium head cauliflower
- 2 tablespoons sesame oil
- 2 cloves garlic, minced
- 1/2 cup diced carrots
- 1/2 cup frozen peas
- 2 green onions, sliced
- 2 eggs, beaten
- 3 tablespoons soy sauce
- Salt and pepper to taste
- Sesame seeds for garnish (optional)

Directions:

- Cut the cauliflower into florets and pulse in a food processor until it resembles rice.
- Heat sesame oil in a large skillet or wok over medium heat.
- Add minced garlic and cook for 1 minute until fragrant.
- Stir in diced carrots and cook for 2-3 minutes until slightly softened.
- Add cauliflower rice and frozen peas to the skillet. Cook for 5-6 minutes, stirring occasionally, until the cauliflower is tender.
- Push the cauliflower mixture to one side of the skillet and pour beaten eggs into the other side.
- Scramble the eggs until cooked through, then mix with the cauliflower mixture.

- Stir in sliced green onions and soy sauce. Season with salt and pepper to taste.
- Garnish with sesame seeds if desired.
- Serve hot.

Tips:

- You can add diced tofu, shrimp, or chicken for extra protein.
- Customize with your favorite vegetables like bell peppers or broccoli.

Chickpea and Vegetable Curry

Preparation Time: 15 minutes

Cooking Time: 25 minutes

Serving Time: Immediate

Total Time: 40 minutes

Ingredients:

- 1 tablespoon coconut oil
- 1 onion, diced
- 2 cloves garlic, minced
- 1 tablespoon grated ginger
- 1 tablespoon curry powder
- 1 teaspoon ground cumin
- 1/2 teaspoon ground turmeric
- 1/2 teaspoon ground coriander
- 1/4 teaspoon cayenne pepper (optional)
- 1 can (15 ounces) chickpeas, drained and rinsed

- 1 can (14 ounces) diced tomatoes

- 1 cup coconut milk

- 2 cups chopped vegetables (e.g., bell peppers, zucchini, carrots)

- Salt and pepper to taste

- Fresh cilantro for garnish (optional)

Directions:

- Heat coconut oil in a large skillet or pot over medium heat.

- Add diced onion and cook until translucent, about 5 minutes.

- Stir in minced garlic, grated ginger, curry powder, ground cumin, ground turmeric, ground coriander, and cayenne pepper (if using). Cook for 1 minute until fragrant.

- Add drained chickpeas, diced tomatoes, coconut milk, and chopped vegetables to the skillet.
- Bring the mixture to a simmer, then reduce heat to low and cook for 15-20 minutes, stirring occasionally, until the vegetables are tender and the flavors have melded together.
- Season with salt and pepper to taste.
- Garnish with fresh cilantro if desired.
- Serve hot with rice or naan.

Tips:

- Customize the vegetables based on what you have on hand or your personal preferences.
- Add a squeeze of lime juice before serving for a burst of freshness.

CHAPTER 5: NOURISHING DINNERS

Baked Salmon with Asparagus

Preparation Time: 10 minutes

Cooking Time: 15 minutes

Serving Time: Immediate

Total Time: 25 minutes

Ingredients:

- 2 salmon fillets
- Salt and pepper to taste
- 1 tablespoon olive oil
- 1 bunch asparagus, trimmed
- 2 cloves garlic, minced
- 1 lemon, sliced
- Fresh dill for garnish (optional)

Directions:

- Preheat the oven to 400°F (200°C).
- Season salmon fillets with salt and pepper.
- Heat olive oil in an oven-safe skillet over medium-high heat.
- Sear salmon fillets skin-side down for 3-4 minutes until golden brown.
- Flip the salmon fillets and add trimmed asparagus to the skillet.
- Scatter minced garlic over the salmon and asparagus.
- Place lemon slices on top of the salmon.
- Transfer the skillet to the oven and bake for 10-12 minutes, or until salmon is cooked through and asparagus is tender.
- Garnish with fresh dill if desired.
- Serve immediately.

Tips:

- Be sure to pat the salmon fillets dry with paper towels before seasoning to ensure a crispy skin.
- Customize with your favorite herbs and spices.

Turkey and Sweet Potato Skillet

Preparation Time: 10 minutes

Cooking Time: 20 minutes

Serving Time: Immediate

Total Time: 30 minutes

Ingredients:

- 1 tablespoon olive oil
- 1 pound ground turkey
- 2 sweet potatoes, peeled and diced
- 1 onion, diced
- 2 cloves garlic, minced
- 1 teaspoon dried thyme
- 1 teaspoon paprika
- Salt and pepper to taste
- Fresh parsley for garnish (optional)

Directions:

- Heat olive oil in a large skillet over medium heat.

- Add ground turkey to the skillet and cook until browned, breaking it apart with a spoon.

- Add diced sweet potatoes, diced onion, minced garlic, dried thyme, paprika, salt, and pepper to the skillet. Cook for 10-12 minutes, stirring occasionally, until sweet potatoes are tender.

- Taste and adjust seasoning if necessary.

- Garnish with fresh parsley if desired.

- Serve hot.

Tips:

- Add bell peppers or spinach for extra vegetables.

- Top with avocado slices or Greek yogurt for added creaminess.

Eggplant Lasagna

Preparation Time: 20 minutes

Cooking Time: 40 minutes

Resting Time: 10 minutes

Serving Time: Immediate

Total Time: 1 hour 10 minutes

Ingredients:

- 1 large eggplant, thinly sliced lengthwise
- Salt for sweating eggplant
- 2 tablespoons olive oil
- 1 onion, diced
- 2 cloves garlic, minced
- 1 pound ground beef or turkey
- 1 can (14 ounces) diced tomatoes
- 1 can (8 ounces) tomato sauce
- 1 teaspoon dried oregano
- 1 teaspoon dried basil

- Salt and pepper to taste

- 2 cups ricotta cheese

- 1/2 cup grated Parmesan cheese

- 1 egg

- 2 cups shredded mozzarella cheese

- Fresh basil for garnish (optional)

Directions:

- Preheat the oven to 375°F (190°C).

- Place eggplant slices on a baking sheet and sprinkle with salt. Let them sit for 15-20 minutes to release moisture.

- Pat the eggplant slices dry with paper towels.

- Heat olive oil in a skillet over medium heat. Add diced onion and minced garlic. Cook until softened, about 5 minutes.

- Add ground beef or turkey to the skillet and cook until browned. Drain excess fat if needed.

- Stir in diced tomatoes, tomato sauce, dried oregano, dried basil, salt, and pepper. Simmer for 10 minutes.

- In a bowl, mix ricotta cheese, grated Parmesan cheese, and egg until well combined.

- Spread a thin layer of the meat sauce in the bottom of a 9x13-inch baking dish.

- Arrange a layer of eggplant slices on top of the sauce.

- Spread half of the ricotta mixture over the eggplant layer.

- Sprinkle half of the shredded mozzarella cheese over the ricotta layer.

- Repeat layers with the remaining ingredients, ending with a layer of shredded mozzarella cheese on top.

- Cover the baking dish with aluminum foil and bake for 30 minutes.

- Remove the foil and bake for an additional 10 minutes, or until the cheese is bubbly and golden brown.

- Let the lasagna rest for 10 minutes before slicing.

- Garnish with fresh basil if desired.

- Serve hot.

Tips:

- You can use store-bought marinara sauce instead of making your own.

- Substitute eggplant with zucchini or sliced mushrooms if preferred.

Lemon Garlic Shrimp Stir-Fry

Preparation Time: 10 minutes

Cooking Time: 10 minutes

Serving Time: Immediate

Total Time: 20 minutes

Ingredients:

- 1 pound shrimp, peeled and deveined
- Salt and pepper to taste
- 2 tablespoons olive oil
- 4 cloves garlic, minced
- 1 red bell pepper, thinly sliced
- 1 yellow bell pepper, thinly sliced
- 1 cup sugar snap peas
- 1 tablespoon soy sauce
- 1 tablespoon honey
- Zest and juice of 1 lemon
- Sesame seeds for garnish (optional)

- Sliced green onions for garnish (optional)

Directions:

- Season shrimp with salt and pepper.

- Heat olive oil in a large skillet or wok over medium-high heat.

- Add minced garlic to the skillet and cook for 1 minute until fragrant.

- Add shrimp to the skillet and cook for 2-3 minutes until pink and opaque. Remove shrimp from the skillet and set aside.

- In the same skillet, add sliced red bell pepper, sliced yellow bell pepper, and sugar snap peas. Stir-fry for 3-4 minutes until vegetables are crisp-tender.

- Return cooked shrimp to the skillet.

- In a small bowl, whisk together soy sauce, honey, lemon zest, and lemon juice.

- Pour the sauce over the shrimp and vegetables. Stir to coat evenly.
- Cook for another 1-2 minutes until heated through.
- Garnish with sesame seeds and sliced green onions if desired.
- Serve hot over rice or noodles.

Tips:

- Customize with your favorite vegetables like broccoli or mushrooms.
- Add a pinch of red pepper flakes for extra heat.

Spaghetti Squash with Turkey Meatballs

Preparation Time: 20 minutes

Cooking Time: 1 hour

Serving Time: Immediate

Total Time: 1 hour 20 minutes

Ingredients:

- 1 spaghetti squash
- 1 pound ground turkey
- 1/4 cup breadcrumbs
- 1/4 cup grated Parmesan cheese
- 1 egg
- 1 teaspoon dried oregano
- 1 teaspoon dried basil
- Salt and pepper to taste
- Olive oil for drizzling
- Marinara sauce for serving

- Fresh basil for garnish (optional)

Directions:

- Preheat the oven to 400°F (200°C).

- Cut the spaghetti squash in half lengthwise and scoop out the seeds.

- Drizzle olive oil over the cut sides of the spaghetti squash and season with salt and pepper.

- Place the squash halves cut-side down on a baking sheet.

- Roast in the preheated oven for 45-50 minutes, or until the squash is tender and easily pierced with a fork.

- While the squash is roasting, prepare the turkey meatballs. In a bowl, mix ground turkey, breadcrumbs, grated Parmesan cheese, egg, dried oregano, dried basil, salt, and pepper until well combined.

- Shape the mixture into meatballs.

- Heat olive oil in a skillet over medium heat. Add meatballs to the skillet and cook for 8-10 minutes, turning occasionally, until browned and cooked through.

- Once the spaghetti squash is done, use a fork to scrape the flesh into strands.

- Serve spaghetti squash topped with turkey meatballs and marinara sauce.

- Garnish with fresh basil if desired.

- Serve hot.

Tips:

- You can use store-bought marinara sauce or make your own.

- Make extra turkey meatballs and freeze them for later use.

Coconut Curry Chicken

Preparation Time: 15 minutes

Cooking Time: 25 minutes

Serving Time: Immediate

Total Time: 40 minutes

Ingredients:

- 1 tablespoon coconut oil
- 1 onion, diced
- 2 cloves garlic, minced
- 1 tablespoon grated ginger
- 2 tablespoons red curry paste
- 1 pound boneless, skinless chicken breasts, cut into bite-sized pieces
- 1 can (13.5 ounces) coconut milk
- 1 cup chicken broth
- 2 cups chopped vegetables (e.g., bell peppers, carrots, broccoli)

- 1 tablespoon soy sauce

- 1 tablespoon fish sauce

- 1 tablespoon lime juice

- Salt and pepper to taste

- Fresh cilantro for garnish (optional)

Directions:

- Heat coconut oil in a large skillet or pot over medium heat.

- Add diced onion and cook until softened, about 5 minutes.

- Stir in minced garlic, grated ginger, and red curry paste. Cook for 1 minute until fragrant.

- Add chicken pieces to the skillet and cook until browned on all sides.

- Pour in coconut milk and chicken broth. Bring to a simmer.

- Add chopped vegetables to the skillet and simmer for 10-15 minutes, or until chicken is cooked through and vegetables are tender.
- Stir in soy sauce, fish sauce, and lime juice. Season with salt and pepper to taste.
- Garnish with fresh cilantro if desired.
- Serve hot over rice or noodles.

Tips:

- Customize with your favorite vegetables and protein like shrimp or tofu.
- Adjust the spiciness by adding more or less red curry paste according to your preference.

Roasted Vegetable Quinoa Bowl

Preparation Time: 15 minutes

Cooking Time: 25 minutes

Serving Time: Immediate

Total Time: 40 minutes

Ingredients:

- 1 cup quinoa
- 2 cups water or vegetable broth
- 2 cups chopped mixed vegetables (e.g., bell peppers, zucchini, carrots, broccoli)
- 2 tablespoons olive oil
- Salt and pepper to taste
- 1 teaspoon dried herbs (e.g., thyme, rosemary, oregano)
- 1/4 cup hummus
- Lemon wedges for serving (optional)
- Fresh parsley for garnish (optional)

Directions:

- Preheat the oven to 400°F (200°C).

- Rinse quinoa under cold water.

- In a saucepan, combine quinoa and water or vegetable broth. Bring to a boil, then reduce heat to low, cover, and simmer for 15 minutes, or until quinoa is cooked and water is absorbed.

- While the quinoa is cooking, spread chopped mixed vegetables on a baking sheet.

- Drizzle olive oil over the vegetables and season with salt, pepper, and dried herbs. Toss to coat evenly.

- Roast vegetables in the preheated oven for 20-25 minutes, stirring halfway through, until tender and lightly browned.

- Divide cooked quinoa among serving bowls.

- Top with roasted vegetables and a dollop of hummus.

- Garnish with fresh parsley and serve with lemon wedges if desired.

- Serve hot or at room temperature.

Tips:

- Use your favorite vegetables or whatever you have on hand.

- Drizzle with balsamic glaze or tahini sauce for extra flavor.

Directions:

- Cut avocados in half, remove the pits, and scoop the flesh into a bowl.
- Mash the avocados with a fork until smooth or chunky, depending on your preference.
- Stir in lime juice, diced red onion, diced tomato, minced jalapeño (if using), and chopped cilantro.
- Season with salt and pepper to taste.
- Serve guacamole with assorted vegetable sticks for dipping.

Tips:

- For extra flavor, add a pinch of cumin or garlic powder to the guacamole.
- Keep the avocado pits in the guacamole to help prevent browning.

Hummus and Whole Grain Crackers

Preparation Time: 5 minutes

Serving Time: Immediate

Total Time: 5 minutes

Ingredients:

- Store-bought or homemade hummus
- Whole grain crackers

Directions:

- Transfer hummus to a serving bowl.
- Arrange whole grain crackers on a serving platter.
- Serve hummus alongside whole grain crackers for dipping.

Tips:

- Garnish hummus with a drizzle of olive oil and a sprinkle of paprika for presentation.
- Experiment with different flavors of hummus such as roasted red pepper or garlic.

Greek Yogurt Dip with Cucumber Slices

Preparation Time: 5 minutes

Serving Time: Immediate

Total Time: 5 minutes

Ingredients:

- 1 cup Greek yogurt
- 1 tablespoon chopped fresh dill
- 1 tablespoon lemon juice
- Salt and pepper to taste
- Cucumber, sliced, for dipping

Directions:

- In a bowl, mix Greek yogurt, chopped fresh dill, lemon juice, salt, and pepper until well combined.
- Transfer the dip to a serving bowl.

- Arrange cucumber slices on a serving platter.
- Serve Greek yogurt dip alongside cucumber slices for dipping.

Tips:

- Add minced garlic or grated cucumber to the dip for extra flavor.
- Sprinkle chopped walnuts or pine nuts on top of the dip for texture.

Mixed Nuts and Dried Fruit

Preparation Time: 2 minutes

Serving Time: Immediate

Total Time: 2 minutes

Ingredients:

- Assorted mixed nuts (almonds, cashews, walnuts, pistachios)
- Assorted dried fruit (raisins, apricots, cranberries, dates)

Directions:

- Combine mixed nuts and dried fruit in a bowl or serving platter.
- Mix well.
- Serve immediately.

Tips:

- Choose unsalted nuts and unsweetened dried fruit for a healthier option.
- Customize the mix with your favorite nuts and dried fruits.

Cottage Cheese and Pineapple

Preparation Time: 2 minutes

Serving Time: Immediate

Total Time: 2 minutes

Ingredients:

- Cottage cheese
- Fresh pineapple, diced

Directions:

- Spoon cottage cheese into a serving bowl.
- Top with diced fresh pineapple.
- Serve immediately.

Tips:

- Use canned pineapple chunks if fresh pineapple is not available.

- Sprinkle toasted coconut flakes on top for extra flavor.

Kale Chips

Preparation Time: 10 minutes

Cooking Time: 15 minutes

Serving Time: Immediate

Total Time: 25 minutes

Ingredients:

- 1 bunch kale, stems removed and torn into bite-sized pieces
- 1 tablespoon olive oil
- Salt and pepper to taste

Directions:

- Preheat the oven to 350°F (175°C).
- Place kale pieces on a baking sheet.
- Drizzle olive oil over the kale and massage it into the leaves until evenly coated.

- Season with salt and pepper.

- Bake in the preheated oven for 10-15 minutes, or until kale is crispy but not burnt.

- Remove from the oven and let cool slightly.

- Serve kale chips immediately.

Tips:

- Customize with your favorite seasonings such as garlic powder, paprika, or nutritional yeast.

- Store leftover kale chips in an airtight container to maintain crispiness.

Apple Slices with Almond Butter

Preparation Time: 5 minutes

Serving Time: Immediate

Total Time: 5 minutes

Ingredients:

- Apples, sliced
- Almond butter

Directions:

- Arrange apple slices on a serving plate.
- Serve almond butter alongside apple slices for dipping or spreading.

Tips:

- Sprinkle apple slices with cinnamon for extra flavor.

- Use peanut butter or any other nut butter
  as a substitute for almond butter.

Berry and Yogurt Smoothie Bowl

Preparation Time: 5 minutes

Serving Time: Immediate

Total Time: 5 minutes

Ingredients:

- 1 cup Greek yogurt
- Assorted berries (strawberries, blueberries, raspberries)
- Granola
- Honey (optional)

Directions:

- Spoon Greek yogurt into a bowl.
- Top with assorted berries and granola.
- Drizzle with honey if desired.
- Serve immediately.

Tips:

- Add sliced bananas or kiwi for extra sweetness and texture.
- Customize with your favorite toppings such as chia seeds, shredded coconut, or nuts.

CONCLUSION

As we reach the final pages of our culinary journey together, it's essential to reflect on the profound impact of embracing a lifestyle centered around nourishing our bodies and revitalizing our health. Through the pages of this cookbook, we've embarked on a transformative voyage toward wellness, guided by the principles of balance, nutrition, and rejuvenation.

As we bid farewell to these recipes, it's evident that they are not merely dishes to be prepared and consumed, but rather tools for empowerment and revitalization. Each recipe within these pages is a testament to the power of wholesome, nutrient-rich ingredients to heal and rejuvenate our bodies from within.

Throughout our exploration of flavors and textures, we've discovered the remarkable ability of food to serve as medicine, particularly in the context of combating fatty liver disease. From vibrant salads bursting with antioxidants to hearty soups brimming with detoxifying herbs, every recipe has been meticulously crafted to support liver health and aid in weight loss.

Yet, beyond the nutritional benefits lies a deeper truth: the act of nourishing ourselves is an act of self-love. In prioritizing our health and well-being, we honor the incredible resilience of our bodies and commit to fostering a harmonious relationship between mind, body, and spirit.

As we close the cover of this cookbook, let us carry forth the lessons learned within its pages into our daily lives. Let us embrace the joy of cooking with intention, savoring each bite as a celebration of vitality and vitality.

May these recipes serve as a constant reminder that true wellness is not merely the absence of illness, but rather a state of vibrant vitality and abundance. And may we continue to nurture ourselves and those we love with the nourishing power of wholesome, delicious food.

In closing, I extend my deepest gratitude to you, dear reader, for embarking on this journey with me. May your kitchen be forever filled with the aromas of health, happiness, and healing. And may your journey towards optimal well-being be as rich and fulfilling as the flavors found within these pages